Home Fitness for Beginners

How to Burn that Fat & Stay Fit at the Comfort of Your Home

By: Seth Andrew McStephen

9781681279572

Publishers Notes

Dedication

To Luna,

Don't give up. Just keep trying.

Table of Contents

Chapter 1 - Know the Importance of Fitness, health & Exercise

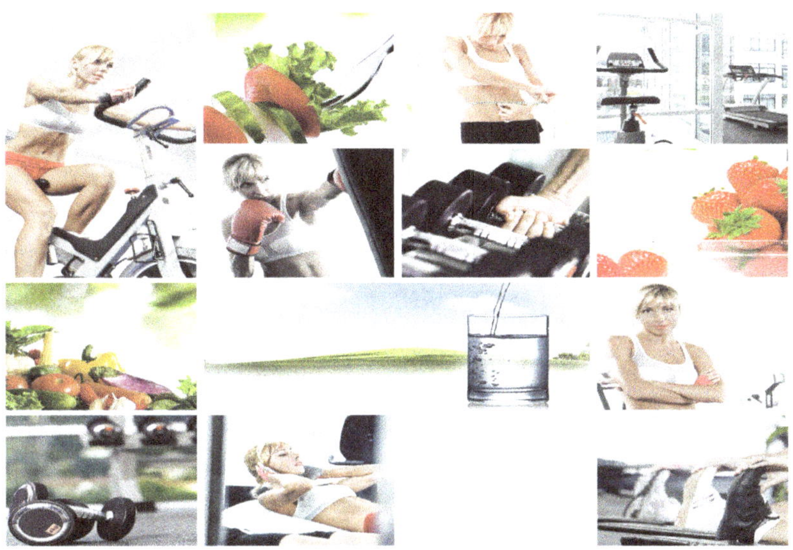

Diet alone is never enough to lose weight and keep it off. Diet alone in fact is never enough to live healthier. Moderate exercises on a timely schedule are imperative for staying fit and healthy, while including a diet with low cholesterol and fat. In fact, most fitness persons misunderstand body fat and cholesterol. Likewise, carbohydrates and calories are also misunderstood.

If you are attempting to lose weight and grow to a healthier living, thus you must understand a few details in order to reach your goals. In the world are all types of people and many suffered illnesses, injuries or other harms that limit their physical activities. Still, these people can exercise in moderation. The experts have provided charts for the injured or ill, helping them to learn how to moderately exercise. Exercise will help us maintain calories, fat, carbohydrates and cholesterol.

Body fats are a requirement of the body, and to determine body fat you must consider that the fat is a percentage the body contains.

Thus, if you weight around one fifty ten percent of the weight is fat. Fat is necessary for the body to function appropriately. Fat controls the body's temperature, while cushions and insulating the tissues and organs. In fact, fat is the chief supporting system for the body to work properly. This is part of the reason that few people exercising and dieting do not grow healthy at times. They plan a diet that cuts out all the fat, cholesterol, carbohydrates, and/or other nutrients the body requires.

On a typical scale, the average person consumes up to 2500 calories each day. Some people exceed the max requirement. Thus, if the metabolism is low, the calories consumed will stick, rather than burn while exercising. Active persons physically fit have less difficulty burning calories.

The energy level then determines the amount of calories a person requires. The basal metabolism rates, which is part of what determines the body's energy level, since the energy exhausted during activities where increased motion is happening, thus the THERMIC food effect also determines the body's energy and how much calories the body will require.

The Basal Metabolic Rates mean that the most of the energy is spent on the body's requirements. Metabolism accordingly is one of the essential factors that determine what the body's weight will reach. The Basal functions or works with the maintenance of the body is temperature, the rate per heartbeats, and the respiration.

When making a goal toward fitness and health by including diet and exercise you will need to know a few details pertaining to fats, cholesterol, carbohydrates and calories. Cholesterol overall is unavoidable. If you consume red meats, margarine, eggs, shrimp, and then you are consuming cholesterol. Once the cholesterol goes in the digestive system and absorbs, it works down to the liver, passing through the circulatory system and finally reaching the blood. Cholesterol produces at its own level in the body naturally, thus excessive consumption will cause the artery walls to clog, which in turn targets the heart, causing death in some instances.

Carbohydrates then are sugars and starches. Thus, high-fibered carbohydrates are not as easily digested as the low-fibered carbohydrates. Yet, Broccoli is one of the high-cellulose, or fibered carbohydrates that have been discovered to reduce hypertension, cancers, arthritis, and diabetes. The low carbohydrates include grains, squash, tomatoes, and cereal. Tomatoes have also been linked to reducing risks of cancer.

Fats are essential for some areas of the body's main function. If you weight around one fifty, thus ten percent of the weight is fat. Calories are also needed to help the body function properly. Few people believe that burning calories is the ultimate method for losing weight, yet, fat, cholesterol and carbohydrates if over consumed can cause the weight to fluctuate, or else cause a person to gain weight with difficulty of losing the weight.

Now to stay fit and healthy while adding a routine of exercises into your plans, you will need to consider the types of foods you digest also. You are what you eat according to few, therefore, be you and watch what you eat.

Important Facts about Being Fit

Exercise is always important, but to keep lean and feel good, there are important facts that you should know about exercising as well. If you are out of shape, you may want to start out a low-moderate exercise routine that lasts for 10 minutes per session to give your body the opportunity to catch up.

You can do 10-minute sessions 3 times per day to get the best results, until you gradually work your way up to 30-minute sessions. One hour is the general rule to quality exercise that creates a lean body. Many types of exercises that you can do to get a lean body, but for the most part, you should learn a bit about the exercises and how each one works to help you avoid harm. If you are just starting out, the last thing you want to do is rush to the gym, workout for an hour, and lift heavy equipment. By doing this type of exercise, you are only asking for trouble. Rather if you are starting out, work with lightweights and low repetitions until your body adjusts.

Your body will let you know when it is ready to move onto heavier weights, and faster repetitions. If you are working out at home, use lightweights with your workout. Cardio workouts are great for firming and toning the body. It also supports the heart muscles, making your heart stronger, which increases your chances of getting a lean body.

Some great aerobic exercises to start are:

- Steps,

- Sit-ups,

- Stretching,

- Flex exercises, and

- Aerobic Dances

Dance aerobics are great since it works the entire body, and you often won't need weights with this type of exercise. You can also start out by walking a few blocks and increasing the blocks as your body adjusts. Stair climbing is another great exercise. You can also wax windows (or even floors without a mop) to work the upper body, and arms. If you practice waxing and stay alert to your motions, you might find your self-learning some karate moves. This is a great secret, which many do not tell you.

One of the best routines found that keeps the body healthy, tone, lean, and feeling good is the series of exercises listed below:

• Always start with the stretch exercises before starting any full workout routine.

• Side stretches four times

• Arm swings four times

• Side stretches two sets

• Elbow lifts two sets eight times

• Side stretches six times

• Elbow Lifts and Torso twist eight times four sets

• Arm swings two times

• Elbow Lift and Torso Twist four sets eight times

• Side stretches eight times

• Arm swings four times

• Reach up

This is a set of exercises that if you follow will start you in the direction to a lean, tone body and a fitness you won't forget.

Next steps

Home Fitness for Beginners

- Head Rolls sixteen times

- Knee Lift and Elbow Touch sixteen times

- Forward Bob and Elbow touch four times

- Forward Lunge and Elbow Touch one time

Repeat the series of steps

Third steps

Side Step

- Toe touches sixteen times

- Rocks thirty-two times

- Toe touches sixteen times

- Hip Twist sixteen times

- Kick and Flick

Sets

- Shake it sixteen times

- Jumping Knee Slaps eight sets

- Shake it sixteen times

- Jumping Knee Slaps eight sets

- Shake it sixteen times

- Jumping Knee Slaps eight sets

- Knee lifts four sets

Fifth Round

- Jumping Knee Slaps eight sets

- Shake it sixteen times

- Knee lifts four sets

- Shake it thirty-two times

- Knee lifts four sets

- Shake it

Know you come to the cool-down where you can relax and stretch the muscles before starting the next round.

- Hold and Point

- Hold and Flex

- Point and Hold eight counts

- Flex and Hold six counts

- Sit-Up-4X

Repeat each series up to the counts and sets you can stand

- Flex Kicks seven sets

Repeat the last series of steps as much as you can stand

Home Fitness for Beginners
Head Tilts seven sets

Shoulder Touches and Elbow Touches ten sets

Continue with two more sets of head tilts

Side Flutter Kicks eighty-eight times

Repeat the last series above for as much as you can stand

Yoga Stretch

Fanny Lifts three and one half times

Single Flex-Kicks eleven times

Repeat the last series.

Chapter 2- How to Start Home Fitness Program

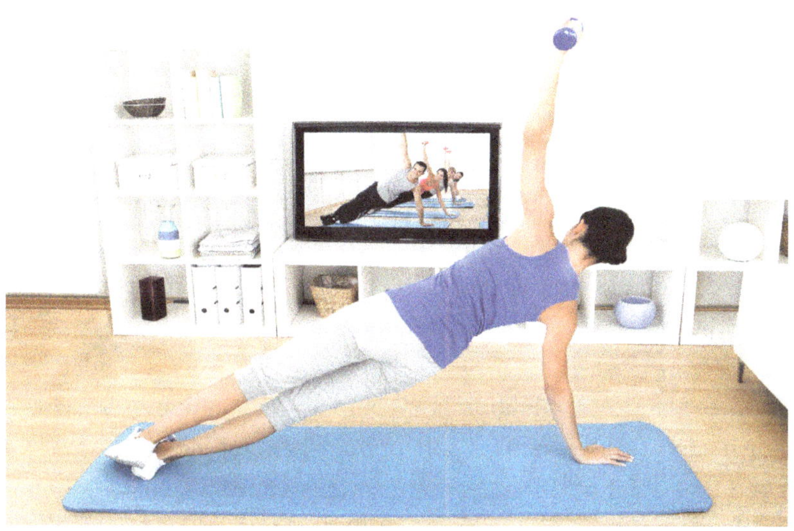

There is one common mistake which many people make when they decide to improve their bodies. This mistake is to not begin with adequate preparation. The first, and most essential, step in preparing to embark on a home workout program is to have a complete health clearance from your physician.

The most important reason for this is you may have a medical problem which you do not know exists. There are many health conditions which can worsen from strenuous exercise; there are some which can even be fatal. While you want to work toward that perfect body, you surely do not want to take unnecessary chances with your health or your life.

An evaluation from your physician will allow you to see if you have any extraordinary risk factors. This kind of check-up, which will take very little time or cost, is well worth the benefits. A clean bill of health will give you peace of mind - and the go-ahead for your home work out.

The second reason is to find out whether you have any special limitations. For example, you may have had sprains or other types of injuries in the past. These can affect choosing the home workout that is right for you. Your doctor may advise you to modify certain kinds of exercise, or to avoid them altogether.

Visiting your physician before you begin a home workout regimen is necessary. If you have any health or medical problems, they need to be addressed before you start a home workout. Anything from a prior injury to an unknown heart condition can prevent you from getting the results you want from your workout. They can cause setbacks and even disaster. A few minutes of your time beforehand can prevent all of this.

The best kind of evaluation is a complete evaluation. If you have not made routine exams a part of your general lifestyle, now is a good time to start. When you are serious about beginning a home workout regimen, you probably already know that it will affect your body. Whether you have exercised before or not, making a home work out a part of your everyday life will place stress and strain on your body. It will affect your muscles, your joints, your blood pressure, and every other part of your system. Your body will be working much harder than it ever did before, to move in the direction of your goals. This is why you need to know in advance that your body is ready for the task. It will help your workouts to proceed more smoothly, and without any unnecessary risks to your health.

A home workout is an exciting adventure. However, in addition to the effects it will have on your body, it will also affect your mind. From the increased blood flow which occurs during workouts, to the change in your blood-sugar levels, the physical benefits of exercise can affect your mood, spirits, and disposition. In order to ensure that these changes are positive and you gain as much from them as possible, you need to be prepared by knowing that you are healthy.

Many people have sustained permanent injuries, and worse, solely due to not being aware of medical problems or limiting conditions prior to starting a regimen of strenuous exercise. Others have become overwhelmed and discouraged, leading them to quit before seeing any positive results. Still others have given up, because they simply did not know what to expect from their new venture. In most cases, all of these repercussions can be avoided.

You want your new home workout routine to produce great results. You want the perfect body that you may have been dreaming of for many years. You want it all to come in the healthiest, safest, and most enjoyable manner, without any unnecessary risks or setbacks. Getting a complete evaluation from your doctor before you choose any exercise or purchase any equipment is the best way to make your home workout routine a positive experience.

When you know that you are healthy, and without any risk factors, you will have a double benefit. First, you can take on the workout routines of your choice without undue risk to your health; and second, you will have the peace of mind from knowing that your new venture is safe for you.

In the interest of your health and safety, make an appointment to see your doctor before you begin your new home workout. Not only is this the most sensible step, it will do wonders for your self-confidence. When you know that you are physically prepared for the home workout routines which you are about to begin, you can look forward to one of the best and most exciting experiences of your life.

Exercise is essential for promoting healthy bones, muscles, reducing health risks, and enforcing the body to function properly. At what time you exercise, some experts tell you to workout outside, since you are getting fresh air. This is a good idea, since fresh air is good, but if you choose to workout inside, make sure you exercise at least one half hour each day.

I do not personally recommend exercising before bedtime, since in my experience, exercise increase the energy level. Unless you are running a marathon in bed, exercising before bedtime is only going to cause you to become restless for a short time.

If you exercise a couple of hours before bedtime, it might work out better, since after a while your body will be tired. It depends on the person, but anyone that exercises regularly can tell you working out before bedtime are not a good idea. Don't be discouraged if after you start an exercise regimen that you find yourself wanting to eat more.

At what time you exercise, it affects your Metabolism. If you find yourself hungry after exercise, wait at least 30 minutes and grab yourself a healthy snack. Sleep disorders or related sleeping problems also include oversleeping. If you find yourself sleeping a lot, it is most likely a direct result of not eating right, and lack of exercise.

Exercise and eating right has proven to be two primary sources for a healthier mind and body. If you sleep a lot, your muscles and bones are affected in a negative way. The more you lie around or sit around the house, the more your bones and muscles will deteriorate. At what time your bones and muscle deteriorate, this soon leads to more complicated health issues. So therefore, whether you sleep too much or do not get enough sleep, part of the solution is to eat healthy, and work those muscles and bones on a daily schedule.

Today, there are hundreds of types of exercises and diets to select from, yet all have their own idea of what the body requires. For example, Carbohydrate pushers lead you to believe that adhering to a CARB diet will give you better results that sticking to other types of diets. Few of these sources fail to tell you that exercise is a requirement of the body. CARB diets are illogical, since the body also requires proteins, fats, carbohydrates, calories, cholesterol, and so on.

If the body is not getting what it requires, regardless of the type of diet you choose, the body will let you down. CARB diets tend to cause a person gain weight as they grow older. Therefore, CARB diets are only an idea that makes someone else money.

The different types of exercises promoted today also hold a bearing on which direction the body will go. If you are doing exercises that do not include covering the entire cardiovascular system, or your routine does not include burning fats or calories, likely you are doing the wrong exercises.

All of us have a different shape of body. The type of exercise then depends on the body type, since some body's work best with mass exercises, while others work best with toning exercises.

Aerobics and weight lifting is one of the better choices of exercises. Combining the two makes it a cross training scheme that is said to work better than merely lifting weights or else participating in aerobics. Still, we have a problem because not everyone can afford to visit a gym.

At home you may not have weights, thus cross training may be out of the question for now. However, the marketplace has few items available for a nominal fee that will help you cross train at home. The steps sold on Television and/or the Internet cost around thirty bucks and will provide you a minimal cross training scheme.

Again, the body has more requirements than merely exercising and dieting. Rather, the requirements include knowing what is right for your type of body. If you start an exercise routine and experience ongoing pain, likely the exercise procedure is not right for your type of body.

Chapter 3- Choosing the Best Home Fitness Program for You

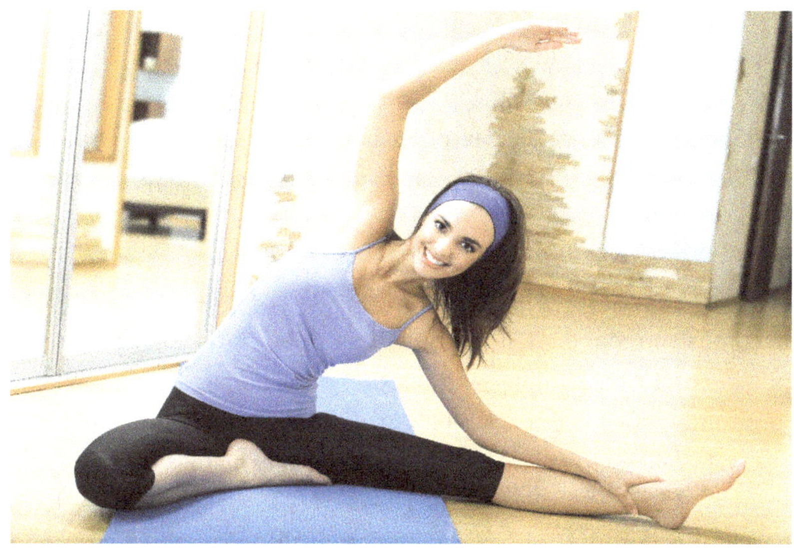

A major change has been observed in the tendency of work out freaks, which is changing their exercise locale from gyms to home. Reason being, the soaring membership prices and binding contracts.

As a result, they have started to opt for home fitness programs. Finding exercises to be done at home is not a complex job, rather a much more convenient option.

There are many great cardio exercises which can be done without much cost to the users. The main money spent is in a good pair of walking, jogging or aerobic shoe, depending on the kind of activity desired.

Besides, a jumping rope is also a great addition for skipping at home because it provides users added alternatives of aerobic workouts that can include rapid work interval training.

Home Fitness for Beginners

One can do it while watching TV or may be by playing music alongside. One should jump for a duration of thirty seconds to a minute as fast as possible and rest in between for sometime before starting again.

You can always perform it during ad commercials and watch the rest of your show calming your body. Today, video and DVD market is flooded with exercise, aerobics and yoga CDs and DVDs which can be purchased for a favorable fitness exercise regime to start at home.

This gives more alternatives to people in case jogging or walking becomes mundane or if the weather does not allow you to go outside and run. Running and walking can actually become all the more interesting if done with a partner, provided no chit-chat and gossip hours begin and win over your fitness schedule.

Varying the ground of the running or walking area can also add change to the daily workout process. Remember, it is very essential that you enjoy what you do to keep yourself fit if you actually want to feel the change in your health and body.

Besides, age does matter while selecting the kind of workout that you do. An adult person may be capable of losing weight using particular equipments and build muscles as well, but an elderly may not just get the same results from the same regimen.

It is simply because of the quality of performance and not the utilization the expensive and similar machines. Thu, it's advisable that you always choose a kind of fitness regimen that goes well with your body, age and needs keeping the various health constraints that age brings along.

Home fitness programs can become as easy or complex as an individual would want to make it from exercises which do not require any additional equipment at all to employing the most advanced fitness gym and aerobic equipments available in the market.

It's beneficial for a person to analyze as to what his goals are for the exercise regime at home and then determine the type of equipments and cost they will charge to accomplish those goals.

Every person has a different body type which makes it essential to find a program that suits every person so that the exercise can be continued for lifetime instead of becoming a passing hobby or fad.

Every person necessitates having some kind of cardio activity included in the workout program, thus different kinds should be tried in order to understand what works for you. Also, it's important to get yourself involved in a physical activity which you can enjoy in the whole fitness program. People who have weak knees, biking are a great option as a home cardio program.

Walking is another low impact cardio physical activity which allows a person to be out while getting workout in his home fitness exercise regime. Cross country skiing and jogging are also two options for those who are more adventurous and those who reside in colder weathers with snow.

Those people who like to employ and can afford equipments for cardio, there are many which can be incorporated in the home fitness programs, like a rowing machine, a treadmill and an elliptical machine. It is better to ascertain as to what exactly are your equipment needs before spending money on them.

Besides, check out for the room where these machines would be placed as some places are not sound enough construction wise to bear such machinery on upper levels. Select the right one for you to get right results.

Home Fitness for Beginners

These days, home workouts are as popular amongst women as they are for men. Women have a natural desire to look and feel their best, too. This is evident by the large number of women who join gyms, purchase exercise equipment, and try various diets. While being more physically attractive and healthier are sensible goals for women, women who wish to begin home workouts do have special circumstances.

One topic is working out during pregnancy. You may have heard "old wives' tales" who claim that no exercise at all is safe when you are pregnant, and you may also heard that virtually nothing is off limits. If you are pregnant, or planning to become pregnant, you may be unsure of which point of view to believe.

With your doctor's approval, working out during pregnancy can be very beneficial. In fact, starting a home workout routine prior to becoming pregnant can prepare your body for this exciting adventure. The better shape your body is in, the easier and more comfortable your pregnancy and childbirth will be for you. It will also make returning to your pre-pregnant state easier and faster after your baby is born.

However, you should be sensible about your home workouts. Your goal is to get your body in its ideal condition, not to overtax your strength or put unreasonable demands on your body. The home workout routine you choose should reflect making your body stronger and more limber, and improving your muscle tone. It is unwise to go to extremes with working out while you are pregnant. If you really want to lift weights, it is best to wait until after your baby is born!

A second topic involves the female anatomy in general. Even when pregnancy is not an issue, you must still take this into consideration. Although it should be obvious, your body is made differently than that of your husband or brother. First, workout routines which place an extreme degree of stress on the abdominal and pelvic regions can indeed cause damage to the internal organs. This is something to keep in mind when you are choosing your home workout program.

In addition, the female muscles are not as prepared for strenuous routines as those of a man's. This does not mean that you cannot obtain the perfect body you want. It does mean taking on less, especially at the beginning, and proceeding slower. If working out is new to you, it is not a good idea to risk tearing muscles by attempting to do too much, too soon.

Whether your body is petite or full-figured, athletic or out of shape, you can have the perfect body of your dreams. In order to avoid the risk of unnecessary injuries, common sense is the key. After all, the purpose of working out is to get your body in its best possible shape, not to incur damage which can slow you down or even become permanent.

The woman who does not have pregnancy as a factor should assess her personal situation before planning a home workout routine. The current condition of your body and how familiar it is with exercise in general, are two points to consider. If you are already athletic, and used to a moderate amount of exercise on a regular basis, you have more leeway than the woman who has never exercised and is quite out of shape.

Thinking about your goals is a positive way to begin. Do you want to increase your overall health, stamina, and be you're most attractive? Firming and toning your body can give you a glowing, youthful appearance, regardless of your age. The body that is strong and fit is also a healthier body. It will reduce your risk of developing many kinds of illnesses and diseases, make everyday life a joy, and can even add years to your lifespan. There is much more to a great body than simply looking good in a swimsuit!

Your goals should be sensible. While you may be able to obtain the body of a female bodybuilder, this is not a common goal for most women. You probably want to get the body you have in its best possible condition, so that you will feel and be more attractive. You probably also want the strong, toned body that reflects good health.

If these are your goals, physical fitness is your answer. You can choose the home workout routines which not only move you toward your goal, but are also much fun to do. Your home workout program will be much more satisfying, and you will be more likely to reach your goals, if you do not start with routines that are too physically-taxing or dull.

Starting with simple routines instead will give you two benefits. First, you will be less likely to incur injury; and second, when you choose fun routines, you will be more likely to continue them faithfully. Your workouts will be something to look forward to, each and every day.

Any woman can have a more attractive, healthier body. Most women can obtain amazing results. The key is to take your circumstances into consideration, and begin your workouts with enthusiasm. You can have that perfect body you have always wanted if you start slowly and proceed with consistency.

Among the number of home fitness programs offered these days, all claiming to be the best and perfect for you. However, not every fitness program presented to you is the best for all. You are a different person with different requirements, lifestyle and wants, thus you cannot have a fitness program which is just meant for all.

Every fitness program comes with its pro's and con's and this is you who will decide that which one suits your needs; you will enjoy, stick to it and also reap full benefits. To help you out, check out an overview of some fitness programs that can adopt at home.

• Aerobics home fitness program

This program comes in many different formats which mainly involve many movements such as leg raises, stretching, arm raises, bending, lunging etc. to music. The frequency and type of movements must depend on your current fitness level. This home fitness program can be followed by using DVD or video on aerobics or even through online sources.

• Pilates home fitness program

In the early 1990's Joseph Hubertis Pilates came with the concept of Pilates which is based on developing and getting better flexibility and body posture of movement originally by utilizing the support of springs. Pilates is practiced by employing specially manufactured equipments or doing exercises that are established on this Pilates system only on a mat. Pilates has produced various versions that are available today on DVD's or videos to be used by you.

• Step fitness home program

Step is mainly a kind of aerobic exercise that involves to step on and off quickly and frequently to music. One can follow this home fitness program by using DVD's or videos at home and a simple equipment piece.

• Dance up a blizzard

Throw on your favorite CD, crank up your music system's volume and dance like a hurricane in your bedroom. Adding more of fun to it can simply have you inviting your friends to come over an indoor house dance party. It can surely be fun for you, your friends and a great way to burn some calories as well. Especially in winters for youngsters and kids, rotating a hula hoop, jumping or juggling rope are easy and fun activities to try inside. Just be certain that you have enough space and high ceilings at your home to avoid damaging any of the furniture.

These are just a few examples of fitness programs that can be done at home. If seriously incorporated in your lifestyle, they can do wonders.

Besides the time factor of gyms mentioned earlier, what about varying your routine for preventing boredom and fitness level? Except for you are ready to spend cash on getting a personal trainer; home fitness program may be just that one appropriate thing that you need.

With extremely quick growth, these programs are becoming popular as the next gen workouts. These programs are divided in three phases for helping you to build lean muscles by utilizing latest innovative circuit training methods. As you will move through every phase, you will notice big changes within 30 days.

Check out few phases for your assistance:

Burn phase- phase 1

The first month when you start with a good home fitness routine your muscles would be pushed to get failure within 10-12 reps focusing on appropriate form that will continue the effectiveness of your workout. Then your routine alters, you avoid fitness and boredom plateaus as you progress to the subsequent phase.

Push phase- phase 2

This is your push phase started in the second month where your muscles would be pushed ahead of its comfort region. The main focus would be on toning each part of your body one at a time to make stronger and also tone every part.

Lean phase- phase 3

This is the last phase called as lean phase where your concentration would be on your body's each part, upper, lower and core. This phase would focus on helping you to get leaner as never before. After surviving the initial two months period, you lose weight, feel great and realize your fullest potential. Further, this provides you with additional energy for achieving your fitness objectives and let you have what you always dreamt of.

Though slowly, but certainly, you get to see your extra weight disappear, lean muscles replacing the extra weight that you use to have. These schedules will fix your metabolism rate on fire and activate your fat burning engines in order to make you burn extra 500 calories every day.

One of the greatest things about the modern day civilization is that there have been a rising number of individuals who are always looking out for ways through which they can be fit and stay healthy.

Besides, the fact that the young generation follows their ideals that are mostly today's celebrity fitness freaks, many along with older people also have started understating the relevance of performing exercises. This has ensured the growth of home fitness programs as well in the times to come.

Chapter 4- Different Types of Aerobic Activity for Everybody

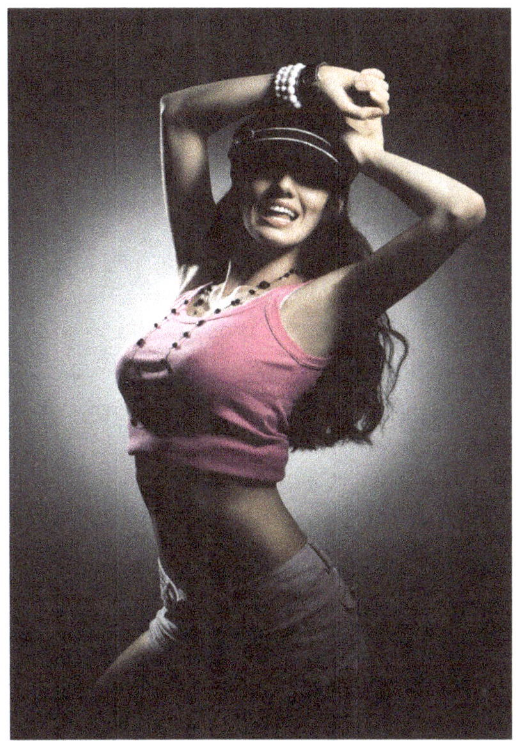

Since Health and Fitness Gyms opened novel aerobic exercises came into play. At the gyms around the world, you can join in Cardio Kick Boxing, Hip Hop Aerobics, Striptease and Martial Arts Aerobics and so on.

Cardio Kick Boxing is comparable to Martial Arts Aerobics, in that it comprises karate into a workout routine... Some of the Martial Arts Aerobics comprise Kick Skills, Choreography, Warm-ups, punches, and so on with each working the complete body.

Striptease Aerobic depend on the trainer, but in few Aerobic Striptease workouts the routine comprises basic spinning, pole dances, transitional and progressive spins, and advanced turn upside down moves. The dance moves could comprise advanced to beginner steps. If you want to become an exotic dancer, this is the aerobics of choice. In fact, this particular aerobics routine was shown on the Oprah Winfrey show. It was brought out in the show that this particular aerobics brings out sexual appeal while toning the body.

If you cannot afford to visit the Gyms, you may want to consider learning home aerobics. The exercises can benefit you, while you work out in the comforts of your home. Few of the fundamental aerobics comprise using the Nordic Track Skier, climbing stairs, jogging around the room, walking in repetition, bicycling, running, canoeing, or using a Video that composes all the steps you need to acquire fitness and health. Most of the aerobics will work the bulky muscles metrically and incessantly, while elevating the hearts rate.

Other exercises including racquetball, tennis, dance, and roller blade and or skating can also enhance your health while you work toward fitness. It is important to check with your physician before starting any aerobic routines and/or other types of exercises.

Nearly everyone running Aerobic classes begin the routines with warm-ups and stretches, while progressively working into a temperate workout. Few instructors will increase velocity following temperate training completion, but few trainers may not. Few trainers are already in to their own routine and fail to see that beginners join their classes. Still, it depends on the instructor. The process of aerobics is intended to amplify the rate of the heart, boost awareness of the body, elevating the body's temperature, and increasing the flow of blood, extending to the muscles.

Aerobics are superior for increasing the heart rate, for restoring the cardio respiratory staying power, while utilizing the larger muscles. Aerobics also enhances the body's composition.

Once you complete a full exercise routine, you will move toward a cool-down workout. It is important to stretch and do warm-ups before aerobics or exercises, as well as cooling down after you finish a routine. The cool-down is intended to reduce the rate of the heartbeats, while averting extreme pooling the blood in the lesser farthest point. Thus, any aerobic routine should include stretches and relaxing workout at the start and completion. The routine helps to shun soreness in the muscles, while enhancing flexibility, and reinstating the balance and/or homeostasis. Furthermore, the cool-down will help to decrease the rate of which the heart beats.

The Hip-hop Aerobics is a boogie aerobic, which combines modern dance with funk. Hip-Hop Aerobics comprises steps that increase energy, while focusing on the entire form of the body. The workout is outstanding for beginners. If you never danced before, perk up those engines because now you will learn to move and groove while working toward fitness and health. If you are trying to lose weight fast, this is the idea aerobics of choice.

The Hi-Lo Aerobic routines work the thighs, heart, abs, calf and so on. Beginners are wise to choice the Hip-Hop or other type of aerobics and work toward this exercise, since it involves rapid movements. The individual moves frequently on one side while slanting in position. The Hi-Lo involves shuffling, turning, shuffling some more, and doubling the knees back while sprinting during the routine and then taking a deep side lunge at speedy pace.

Funk and Jazz Aerobics comprise low-impacting workouts, which generally include jazz steps, funk twists and yoga. Some include the PILATE aerobics, but mostly the exercise is great for newcomers into the gym, since no heavy gear is involved. The routine is generally temperate.

Boogie Aerobics

Aerobic dances have been fashionable in the past few years. In the precedent decades, fitness and health centers have grown, extending on their routines and weight ideas offered. Most health and fitness clubs present an assortment of exercises, including weight lifts, PILATES, yoga, aerobics, spinning, kick boxing, karate, and more.

The selection of health and fitness clubs frequently have their own exclusive styles to assist individual's in losing weight, increasing muscle mass, toning the bodies, strengthen the bones and so on. Aerobic exercises have tempting headings intended to catch the eye. The titles include the Hi-Lo aerobics, Aerobics rooted on Martial Arts, Aerobic Striptease, Cardio Kick Boxing, Hip-Hop, Funk and Jazz, and so on. Some of the aerobic routines include equipment to enhance exercise and fitness experiences.

Slide or Step Aerobics implicates equipment. During the Step Aerobics routines, you position a footstep in the frontage, which you step one foot up, down and up on the other leg, replicating the course of action for quite a few minutes. The process is intended to tone the lower body; still concerns of Step Aerobics have made statements, since the ankles and knees are normally utilized often. The Slide Aerobics involves a step, and in its place of stepping up repetitiously to the frontage, the work outer steps to the side, slide downward, and then slides back up. The Slide Aerobics show a discrepancy in each Health and Fitness Gyms. Some Slide Aerobics might implicate equipment, including the Nordics Ski.

Before joining a Health and Fitness Club, make sure you are aware of the types of aerobics offered to you, since few clubs might offer more affective aerobic courses than others will. Some clubs have trainers available willing to help you choose the right aerobics for you, while other clubs merely want their pay. For example, some clubs may offer aerobic routines that focus on flexibility. The aerobic routines will mostly involve stretches, which means you will not receive the results you are possibly searching to achieve, including losing weight fast.

Hi-Lo Aerobics flowing

Hi-Lo Aerobics involves a fast-paced routine that includes rapid movement. The individual moves typically on the side and in a slanting position. During the Hi-Lo you will shuffle, turn, shuffle, and double the knee back, while sprinting during, and taking a profound side lunge at swift paces. The Hi-Lo aerobics work the Calf, Thighs, Abs, Heart Legs, and so on. Beginners would benefit more by choosing a different type of aerobics exercise, since the Hi-Lo is more for the advanced. The main idea of aerobics is not hurting your self-while better your health.

Hip-hop Aerobics is a dance routine, which mix together funk with contemporary dance. The Aerobic dance implicates the usage of high-energy dance, while working out the complete body. The work out is optional, but works for everyone. If you are a novice who knows nothing about dancing, do not fret, as the instructor will direct you through the process; include teaching you the grooves, rhythm, rhyme and moves. If you are training to lose weight, the Hip-Hop is a first-class alternative to decide on, since dance has proven to be one of the most effective exercises to date.

Funk and Jazz aerobics depend on the Fitness and Health Center, as to what the Aerobics include, but few clubs merge low-impact work out that often includes exhilarating jazz dances with a twist of funk and yoga. Funk and Jazz is an option for beginners, since the training does not include weighty equipment and the routines are temperate.

Cardio Kick Boxing relies on the trainer, but mainly Cardio Kick Boxing is an elevated work out for getting in shape promptly, while learning techniques to perk up physical robustness. The work out includes footwork while merging karate kicks and strikes. Cardio helps you to lose weight, tone the body, increase muscle, while teaching self-defense. Cardio Kick Boxing frequently comprises jump rope, crunches, stretches, bag punches, kicks, and pushups.

Dance Aerobics for the Beginners

Dance aerobics include steps, funk, and powering the rump. Persons that lack the artistic ability to dance may wonder why join a class that includes dancing. The trainers at most gyms have made it convenient for beginners to take the front in aerobic dance steps. The aerobics will tone the body, add volume, increase flexibility, and enforce staying power.

While you might find it difficult to learn that steps to perfection at first, in time, you will learn, but in the meantime, you are burning off those calories. When the body sweats because of movement, the calories start to burn, which in turns reduces pounds.

After joining a class, you will quickly learn why continuing dance aerobics is smart. The dance aerobics is the better option for increasing the hearts muscle, while increasing oxygen levels at the same time. Dance aerobics enhance metabolism, while improving balance.

After getting started, your body will take you, since it will feel great. Aerobics that include dance steps may entail stepping forward on one foot, while raising the knees simultaneously on the other leg. One other well-known step in aerobics that includes dance steps is marching in place. Overall, it is vital that you learn minimal details pertaining to the exercise, including what gear to wear, which will include shoes and clothes.

Other steps in dance aerobics include spinning, twirling, and moving the feet in motion to the beat. Since dance aerobics not only involves dancing in place, it is important that you wear that appropriate attire and shoes. If you fail to adhere to advice, the dance aerobics might end up being an uncomfortable routine. Avoiding the right attire and shoes can also lead to injury.

The body sweats during any workout. Therefore, wearing fitting clothes is essential when dancing. Weightless clothes are the choice, since it helps while you sweat, and the right clothes can support breasts, especially for women. Jocks are recommended if men are joining dance aerobics.

While participating at your first dance class, it is wise to show up at least fifteen minutes early. Instructors are available during training, and if you show up early, the instructor can learn your status in the club. The instructor can spend a few minutes, to make sure you are spotted appropriately.

If you are a beginner, it is advised that you participate in dance aerobic classes that start with basic dance steps. The classes that employ the Hi-Lo dance moves are the best option for beginners. The step-funk and power the rump classes are more for the advanced trainers, thus if you cannot dance, this is not idea for you.

Dancing is an art, which requires mastering overtime. Some people require experience, while others learn rapidly. Few of the better dancers on Television start out as novice dancers, and few did not have a starting point. Once you get into the groove however, learning a few moves, it shouldn't take long to learn a few more steps. If you are not dance oriented, this too will become noticeable.

If large crowds make you, nervous you may want to pay attention at the mirrors located in the Gym. The mirrors are often attached to the walls, and surround the entire workout area. Consequently, if you are anxious at what time you walk in the entrance, it might be to your advantage to watch the mirrors and avoid looking at the trainers. Make certain that you keep an eye on the instructor so that you do not fail to spot steps. An alternative, is following this priceless tip and avoid putting too much forethought into what the trainer is saying. Instead, put more scrutiny into what the trainer is doing. This will facilitate in decreasing anxiety.

In time, you will learn the steps in dance aerobics if you apply self. Exercises, especially those that work with the cardiovascular system, muscles and bones are the best form of exercises available. Dance in my experience, is one of the better choices of exercises that helps keep the body tone, firm, while maintaining weight.

Aerobics Cross Training Basic

Aerobics involve using the large muscles incessantly while moving the body in rhythmically motion. The routines enhance beats of the heart and smoothest the breathing repetitions. Full body aerobic exercises might comprise the basics, including dance, walking in place, ski, bicycling, running in place and jogging. It is important to learn about the aerobics before starting routines to avoid injury.

The objective is important before starting aerobics. Once you know your objective, you will know what you want from the exercises. You should also consider the condition of your health, including genetics and history of disease in the family. Preceding injuries should also be considered before starting aerobics.

To get started, what is your objective? Is your goal to lose weight and/or burn fat? If you have a goal in mind and it is to burn fat and lose weight considering your goal, health and history can help you avoid injury during workout and harm to injuries from the past. Cross training then, is one of the better choices of aerobics to prevent injuries. Cross training is merely combining one aerobic routine with another routine, such as half weights and aerobics. Cross training will help you achieve equilibrium of training schedules.

Before considering cross training however, we must understand the different exercises. Few exercises include the low-temperate workouts, high-impact workouts, and so on. If you are intending to lose weight and burn fat, combining the low and high-impact aerobics together can give you faster results. For example, if you include low-temperate aerobics with high-impact aerobics you might walk, step, ski, dance, run, or play racquetball. The idea timeframe is three to five days each week and at least one hour each set.

The mixture reduces risk especially if you suffer from preceding or present injury, including hip injury, low back injury, ankle, or other related injuries. If you have existing injury the experts tell you to workout in moderation, this is why it is important to consult with your doctor before starting aerobic routines. Most likely, the doctor will tell you to avoid ski exercises if you had prior injuries.

Cardiovascular exercise are intended to make available complete body augmentation while strengthen the muscles and bones. Of course, this includes strengthening of the joints, while reducing fats and calories. The cardio workouts will help develop muscles and boost Cardiovascular. Working out can enhance the body's flexibility as well. As you can see the correct cross-training routines is essential. If you are considering high-impact workouts, such as running you may want to combine bicycling, stretches and weights at least once each week. The combo will strengthen the muscles, while enhancing the body.

If you considered jogging, then it can enhance the fitness, while improving cardio. Jogging includes using the large muscles; however, the problem is that it will not increase mass also. Cross-training then will include working the upper body, which may include weights, or correct aerobics that work the upper body. In spite of everything, you are not acquiring flexibility, which the body demands. To include cross training exercises for flexibility, include stretching and warm-ups into your routine.

Experts of sport have claimed that cross training is one of the better choices, since it provides constructive results. Combing exercises is the hit of the higher points in physical working out. Summing it up, cross-training exercises if choosing the correct combination, will burn fat, strengthen muscles and bones, reduce calories, and produce flexibility, while working the complete body. Cross training can lend a hand to individuals trying to build up the body. Cross training can also make available sources of pleasure, as well as enhancing energy levels, which includes building Metabolism.

If your goal is to acquire fitness, then you are required to comprise strength walking, vigorous walking, swim, jog, ski, bicycle riding, skating and other types of exercises into your routine. To strengthen the muscles use free weights, or isometric workouts. Isometric workouts are opposite muscle workouts that contract since it includes minuscule restraints but boost in tone of muscle fibers. It is important to keep fit if you want good health, therefore learn the right cross training steps for you.

CHAPTER 4- BENEFITS OF HOME FITNESS

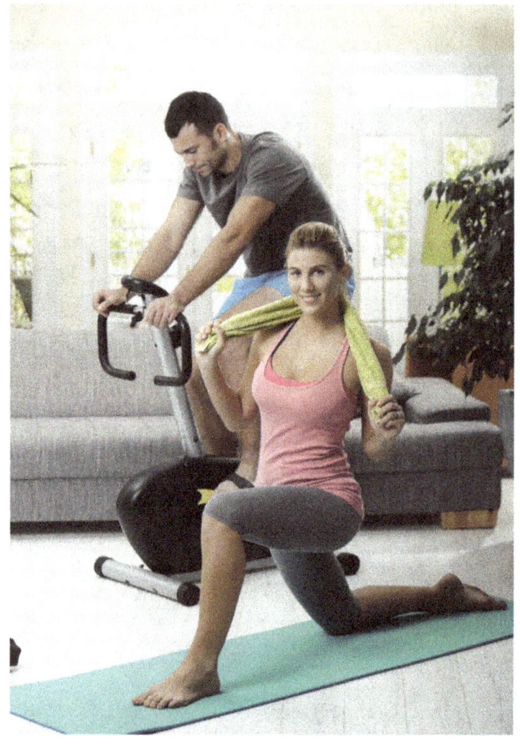

Home fitness programs provide many benefits to those people who want to do workout but have less time and desire of going to a gym. However, a major aspect of home fitness programs comes with its privacy facility.

Especially people who feel awkward to work out in front of others because of many reasons such as self esteem hesitation etc. Also, you do not have to dress up to get ready for going to a gym as you would be working out at home.

You can wear anything you want without worrying about what others might think. Besides, you won't need to worry about doing a particular exercise wrongly and embarrass yourself.

Everything is under your control, you can mess up the number of times you want to and no one would get to know. There would be no need of looking for women's only or men's only sections as home based health regime is your own private arena where you can be as comfortable as you always wanted.

Also, you get to work out at your own speed, the way you want to utilize your equipment at your home. There can't be a much easier and better option for you than this which also saves your money that you spend on gym membership and on gas for driving to it.

So many times an occurrence exists when you are not well for long number of days and do not go to your gym. However, your money keeps on getting deducted at your gym. By investing in your home fitness program, you not just attain ease and health but also lifetime assets for continuing with fitness.

Today, people of every age put fitness as their major priority, but this does not mean everyone can afford to bear the hefty costs of gyms to respect this priority. This is why; there are many other home fitness program alternatives that can be adopted by teenagers who are most of the times short of money.

Running or jogging on the streets won't cost you anything but just lend you ample amount of positive energy and good health. Even getting two or three gym equipments for yourself is a better idea, saving you from the annual or half yearly gym membership costs.

Leaving you with no excuses to avoid exercising outside, home fitness programs are one of the best things to invest in today because every individual needs to be healthy today to have a happy future tomorrow!

Leaving you with no excuses of not finding the right type of exercises that you can do at home, here is a list of the appropriate home fitness based program exercises for you.

● These exercises can be performed by using easy drills at home and employing minimal equipments which you can get from around your house.

● For upper body you can do chair dips, lateral raises, push-ups, chin ups and bent over row. For core exercises you can do dead

lift, sit ups and Side Bridge.

● For lower body you can opt for step ups, wall squat, bucket squats and lunges. Prior to starting these exercises you must warm up yourself for minimum of five minutes by jogging or brisk walk around the block or by skipping on the spot. You must perform multiple sets of the exercises mentioned above depending upon your endurance level and requirement.

Also, taking intervals in between is equally essential. You can combine two exercises that use diverse muscle groups alternating between two things that provide each muscle group some rest while you perform another.

To get the best results, perform these workouts at least thrice a week, with no less than a day between exercises for sufficient recovery. You must always strive to increase the intensity or load and to increase your fitness growth.

Once your fitness improves, you can undergo this routine without bothering much and start with a more superior program. Use your creativity and find more things to use for working out at home. Using buckets, filled with the amount of water you want can be employed for squats and step ups.

Filling up milk bottles with 2 liter water makes it equivalent to a 2 kg weight to be used for overhead triceps extension, bicep curls and bent over rows. Shopping bags and backpack filled with items can be used for lunges, step-ups and squats.

Utilizing bricks by breaking them in half in case of lower weight is appropriate for pushups, bench press, lateral raises and front raise. Then, the age old forms of exercises that come under the practice of yoga asana. A lot of people not just perform these exercises for the sole aim of relieving mental stress but to get and stay fit as well.

If you look at the fitness regimens of every famous celebrity today including the big names like Jennifer Aniston, Drew Barrymore, it is yoga that has worked wonders on their body to get the envious figure every girl wants. Not only women, even men have also started incorporating this form of fitness to build up muscles using their own body weight. This is the most natural way of dealing with your body and respecting it as well.

Chapter 5- Important Advice From the Experts

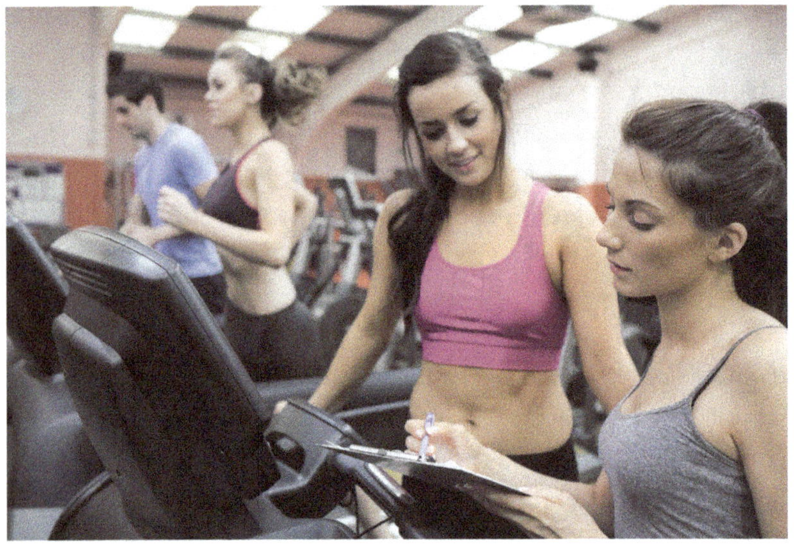

Experts are continually learning innovative particulars regarding the body, nevertheless, the information accessible concerning body types is a foundation to relating to the type of body, which assists in determining which diet plans work paramount to your body type.

When consider body type one should stay alert to the types of exercises that suit the body type best. The hormones are essential when considering exercises. The hormones are chemical dispatch riders, which send communiqué to the electrical system within the body. The electrical system is also known as the Central Nervous System (CNS), which includes the brainpower.

The hormones decide on the person's thoughts, feelings, and how a person will develop according to the experts. The body composes cells, nerve endings, nuclei, which are a cluster of chemicals produced in brain cells, glands, and various other organs, which influence a huge number of functionalities within the body.

Hormones producing such chemicals only drop or raise the aging process. The hormones will determine the amount of pain and anguish our health will endure, as well as affecting the metabolism, while deciding on the body's mass, or weight. The hormones indirectly or directly affect the person's height, perception, memory, blood pressure, digestion system, just to name a few.

Hormones send chemicals to the endocrines gland, which the consequences is the secreting of hormone dispatching in to the bloodstream. The affect is that the body's functional system of cells and other organ's affect the entire body. Thus, the CNS also plays a large role in the changes our body accepts.

As you can see, the body requires balance. Balance is part of losing weight. The Endomorph then is a body type that often has large bones, huge trunk area, spherical face, and thighs, which has a lot of body fat biologically. The body fat on this type is often found near the midsection, which means these types of body's fight back to preserve weight or else lose weight.

The Endomorph body type demands motivations higher than the MESOMORPH AND ECTOMORPH types. This is necessary to maintain weight. Thus, burning fat, increasing metabolism, and including low-intense exercises combined with high-endurance exercises is the idea combo for this type of body, yet devoid of over training.

Endomorph bodies tend to work best at the lesser objective heart rate precinct. The body requires oxygen, which must flow smoothly to increase your health and reduce the weight, or maintain a weight level.

Once the body develops or adjusts, you will need to increase the volume of exercises. The endomorph types are told to reduce the caloric intakes, while consuming an abundance of low caloric provisions.

MESOMORPH types are more of the bodybuilding types. The MESOMORPH body can enjoy high-intense weight lifting with ease, while enjoying temperate aerobics.

The MESOMORPH body has larger bones and thicker skin, thus dieting should include low-fat provisional foods, with advanced caloric intake. The MESOMORPH body often pans out as the body decreases fat intake and increases calorie intakes, providing the person conform to regular workout schemes.

The ECTOMORPH type has lower body fat, with high volumes of mass. These types are said to suffer repeated hot flashes, since the fat in the body is lacking. The ECTOMORPH types require more fatty foods to maintain a level of weight, and an extreme intake of calories than other types.

The ECTOMORPH has difficulty gaining weight, thus the body requires heavy weight lifts with increasing repetitions after the body adjusts. The hormones playing a large role, brings us to the point. Regardless of the body type, we all have hormones, which mean we need a balanced diet and proper exercises to promote hormonal producing, endomorph producing, and other productions that the body demands.

With this in mind you also want to consider Glycogen and Oxygen, which both play a major part in weight gain or lose. While experts all have their idea as to what keys in to good health and fitness, it is up to us to find what works best for our body. Cross training is said to be one of the better solutions for burning fat, reducing calories, losing weight, building strength and so on.

According to few insulin levels play the largest role in losing weight. Other experts determine that our body type is the key to finding the proper exercises and diet plans that work with the body.

To achieve a healthier status and maintain weight diet must combine with exercise, since one without the other will not work. Combining healthy provisions with correct exercises can bring you good health and physical fitness, which will enhance your quality of life. It will also help you keep your body's zone to a level.

The body and mind is complicated, however both work together to produce results. Many experts, including theorists, doctors, scientist, and philosophers are continuing to find answers to the body's functions.

Some of the confusion comes when people diet, exercise and take care of them self, yet they still gain weight. Barry Sears wrote a compelling book titled A Week in the Zone, which produced some outstanding advice. Some of the information in the book helps us to decide on exercises and diets that suit us best, since insulin plays a large part in healthier living.

The author lets us know that the hormones consequence of intakes of carbohydrates and caloric differ from the hormones that produce protein and calories. , he continues letting us know that the effects of hormones that produce fats and calories too differ in the direction of health.

The author brings us to see that a balance is needed, yet the balance is factored by the different hormonal levels. Thus, eating healthy, giving the body proper fluids and exercising is the only answer to living a productive and quality lifestyle.

One of the biggest setbacks that people adhere to is making excuses to avoid dieting and exercise. Countless of people find it easier said than done to stick with diet and exercise programs that facilitates them to remain healthy while maintaining weight.

One of the largest reasons is that most people do not understand their body and its type, or have difficulty adhering to a schedule.

One of the largest reasons why this happens is that many people find it difficult to plan, set goals that work, and find solutions that help the person maintain a schedule. The threesome is the ultimate tools for working toward good health and fitness.

If you are uncertain of the types of exercises, this too can hold you back. Walking up and down the stairs is an aerobic exercise. Mowing the lawn is another type of exercise. Anytime the body is in motion, producing actions it is exercising. Lifting 12' ounces of beer is not an exercise. Alcohol if overused will affect the body and mind dramatically.

Other forms of exercise are merely walking to the store instead of driving your car, especially if the store is down the road. If you find it, difficult getting started with exercise makes effort to ask a friend or family member to join you. Otherwise, possibly at your workplace a team of people is joining a gym to better their health, maybe you can go with them. If you have a dog, dogs enjoy walking, therefore put your feet in motion and make your dog happy. Children also enjoy walking with parents, therefore spend time with your children and exercise while doing so.

Therefore, if you have intricacy with setting goals, planning, or sticking to a schedule, begin by using the stairs in place of an elevator at what time you visit your doctor, or other appointments. In addition, you could scythe the lawn in place of paying the fellow citizen down the street to do the work for you. Beginning exercise is by no means easy, but you have to start somewhere to reach a healthier status!

ABOUT THE AUTHOR

Seth Andrew McStephen is a personal trainer and all round lover of exercise and fitness. After being bullied as a child because of his weight, he decided to make a change and he dedicated all of his spare time into getting fit and losing weight. In his books including the "Home Fitness for Beginners: How to Burn that Fat & Stay Fit at the Comfort of Your Home" he brings the world of home fitness to the public, and gives them a glimpse into this convenient world. He lives in LA, with his beautiful wife and his Pug, Stan.